BORON THE MIRACLE CURE

"Unveiling The Ultimate Power of Letter B Element"

Shanika Steve

Table of Contents

CHAPTER 1 ....**5**

Introduction...5

What is Boron? 6

CHAPTER 2 ....**9**

Importance of Boron in the Body **9**

Bone Health 9

Hormonal Regulation 10

Brain Function 12

Immune System Support 14

CHAPTER 3 ....**17**

Boron Deficiency...**17**

Causes of Boron Deficiency 17

Symptoms of Boron Deficiency 18

CHAPTER 4 ....**21**

The Role of Boron in Health and Disease..........**21**

Arthritis and Joint Health 21

Osteoporosis Prevention 22

Menopausal Symptoms Relief 24

Cognitive Function Enhancement..................... 26

Antimicrobial Properties 27

CHAPTER 5 ....**30**

Food Sources of Boron.................................**30**

CHAPTER 6 .... **35**

Boron Supplements **35**

Creating a Brain-Healthy Environment 35
Types of Boron Supplements............................ 36
Safety Considerations 37

CHAPTER 7 .... **40**

Potential Risks and Side Effects of Boron **40**

Conclusion... **45**

CHAPTER 1

Introduction

The body requires the trace mineral boron. Despite being frequently disregarded in comparison to other minerals like calcium or iron, boron is essential for several physiological processes. Boron is engaged in a wide range of processes that improve general health, from promoting bone health and hormone regulation to improving brain activity and immune system response.

The significance of boron in the body, the effects of boron shortage, and the potential advantages of ensuring a proper intake of this mineral are all covered in this detailed book. We will also review boron supplements, evaluate the daily suggested dosage, and look into food sources that contain this element. We will also discuss any possible hazards or negative consequences of boron usage.

For anyone looking to maximize their wellbeing, understanding the role of boron in health and disease is essential. This manual will give you useful information whether you're interested in preserving healthy bones, reducing menopausal symptoms, promoting cognitive function, or learning more about boron's antibacterial characteristics.

By the conclusion, you will have a better grasp of the role that boron plays in the body and how it can improve a number of different elements of your health. Even though boron appears to have promising benefits, it is always best to speak with a healthcare provider before making any significant dietary or supplemental changes.

So let's go out on this adventure to learn about the various advantages and treatments of boron and see how this sometimes ignored mineral might improve your general health and wellbeing.

What is Boron?

Chemically speaking, boron has an atomic number of five and the letter "B" in its periodic table. Given that it is a metalloid, it possesses both metallic and nonmetallic qualities. Naturally occurring borates, which are boron compounds with oxygen and other elements, are the most common form of boron found in the Earth's crust.

Boron is a solid that is either dark brown or black when it is pure. Borax, kernite, and ulexite are a few examples of the several borate minerals that are more frequently found in the environment. With major concentrations found in nations including the United States, Turkey, Chile, and China, these minerals are widely scattered throughout the Earth's crust.

Since ancient times, people have employed boron for a variety of purposes. Borax, a substance containing boron, was utilized in the past in the creation of glazes and ceramics, giving rise to its application. Currently, boron is used in many different sectors, such as glass production, ceramics, detergents, agriculture, and nuclear reactors as a neutron absorber.

The trace mineral boron is regarded as crucial for biological processes. Accordingly, even though the body only needs tiny amounts of boron, it is essential for boron to play a vital role in preserving optimal health and functioning. In particular, bone health, hormone regulation, brain function, and immune system support are among the physiological processes in which boric acid is engaged.

In recent years, there has been a growing interest in learning more about the role of boron in the body and potential medicinal uses for the element. Boron's potential as a beneficial nutrient and therapeutic agent is being revealed by researchers as they continue to study its effects on all facets of health and disease.

The specific functions of boron in the body, the effects of boron shortage, and the advantages of ensuring a proper intake of this crucial mineral will all be covered in more detail in the sections that follow.

CHAPTER 2

IMPORTANCE OF BORON IN THE BODY

Bone Health

One of the important functions of boron in the body is its role in supporting strong bones. When it comes to bone metabolism, boron is essential because it affects how other essential minerals, including calcium, magnesium, and vitamin D, are absorbed and used.

Boron supplementation may improve bone health by raising bone mineral density (BMD) and lowering the risk of osteoporosis, according to a number of studies. Low bone mass and bone tissue degeneration are the hallmarks of osteoporosis, which increases the risk of fractures.

It is thought that the action of boron on important biochemical processes involved in bone development and maintenance is what causes it to have such positive effects on bone health. It is believed to increase the synthesis of testosterone and estrogen, two hormones essential for controlling the metabolism of bones. Boron may aid in maintaining bone density and lowering the incidence of fractures, especially in postmenopausal women, by boosting the manufacture of these hormones.

Additionally, boron appears to improve calcium and magnesium absorption and usage, two minerals crucial for bone health and structure. Boron may help to maintain strong bones and stop bone loss by increasing the availability and use of these minerals.

While boron has the potential to enhance bone health, further research is required to determine the best dosages, the best period for supplementation, and the usefulness of boron in various groups. As with any dietary or supplement modifications.

Hormonal Regulation

The body's hormonal system is significantly regulated by the element boron. It has been demonstrated to have an impact on the synthesis, metabolism, and action of a number of hormones, including testosterone, estrogen, and vitamin D.

The levels of physiologically active estrogen, which are crucial for preserving reproductive health and general hormonal balance, have been observed to rise in both men and women when boron is present. As boron supplementation has been linked to relief from menopausal symptoms like hot flashes, night sweats, and vaginal dryness, it is especially advantageous for postmenopausal women.

Boron has been linked to higher testosterone levels in men. A vital hormone for male reproductive health, muscle growth, and bone density is testosterone. According to studies, men who use boron supplements may have higher amounts of free testosterone, the hormone's biologically active form, which may boost their libido and general vigor.

Additionally, vitamin D, a hormone necessary for calcium absorption, bone health, and immune system performance, is activated by and processed by boron. According to some research, boron helps vitamin D become active, boosting the vitamin's positive effects on bone metabolism and general health.

Researchers are still looking into the precise methods through which boron affects hormone synthesis and metabolism. However, it is thought that boron may interfere with hormone receptors in the body and disrupt the enzymes responsible for hormone synthesis and metabolism.

Brain Function

It has been discovered that boron may offer advantages for cognitive health and brain function. According to research, boron may contribute to improved cognition in general, including memory and attention.

Studies on both humans and animals have produced encouraging findings in regards to the benefits of boron supplementation on cognition. Boron appears to affect synaptic activity and neurotransmitter activity, both of which are necessary for healthy brain function. According to some theories, boron may improve cognitive function by encouraging the release and usage of important neurotransmitters like dopamine and serotonin.

Boron has also been shown to shield the brain from oxidative stress and inflammation. Cellular harm can result from oxidative stress, which is brought on by an imbalance between free radicals and antioxidants in the body. It also plays a role in neurological illnesses like Alzheimer's and Parkinson's. The antioxidant qualities of boron may lessen oxidative stress and inflammation, thereby defending the health of the brain.

The data points to boron's potential as a neuroprotective agent and cognitive enhancer, even though the precise mechanisms by which it influences brain function are still not completely understood. To determine the best dosages, long-term effects, and precise demographics that would benefit the most from boron supplementation, more research is nonetheless required.

While boron appears to be beneficial for maintaining brain health, it should be noted that neither cognitive decline nor neurodegenerative illnesses may be cured by boron. For overall brain health, it's still important to maintain a healthy lifestyle that includes a balanced diet, regular physical activity, mental stimulation, and enough sleep.

The significance of boron in boosting the immune system and its possible advantages for immunological function and infection protection are discussed in the next section.

Immune System Support

The immune system, which is in charge of protecting the body from pathogens and preserving general health, is supported by boron. Numerous studies have revealed that boron may have positive impacts on the immune system, despite the fact that the precise mechanisms underlying these effects are not yet fully understood.

According to research, boron may promote the growth and function of some immune cells, including lymphocytes and natural killer cells. These cells play a crucial role in the body's immune response because they assist in locating and getting rid of dangerous infections and infected cells.

Boron's ability to regulate cytokine synthesis and activity, signaling molecules involved in controlling immunological responses, may be the cause of its ability to modulate immune function. Pro-inflammatory cytokines, which are necessary for generating a successful immune response to infections, have been discovered to be affected by boreon.

The immune-boosting benefits of boron may also be a result of its antioxidant qualities. Boron may help the immune system work more effectively and improve the body's capacity to fight off infections by lowering oxidative stress and inflammation.

The depth of boron's effects on immune system support requires further study, but the information that is already available points to boron's potential as a beneficial nutrient for general immune health. To maintain a healthy lifestyle, which includes a balanced diet, regular exercise, stress management, and enough sleep, which is still essential for optimum immune function, it is vital to keep in mind that boron supplementation should not be viewed as a stand-alone treatment for immune-related problems.

The effects of a boron shortage and the potential advantages of ensuring an appropriate intake of this crucial mineral for numerous areas of health and disease are discussed in the sections that follow.

CHAPTER 3
BORON DEFICIENCY

Causes of Boron Deficiency

Humans rarely have boron deficiencies since boron intake is often very low. However, there are a few things that can make the body's boron levels insufficient. The following are some potential reasons for boron deficiency:

1. Poor dietary intake: Boron shortages are most frequently caused by a diet lacking in boron-rich foods. Generally speaking, plant-based foods such as fruits, vegetables, legumes, nuts, and some grains contain the most boric acid. The risk of boron deficiency may be higher in people who consume a diet that is high in processed foods but low in fresh produce.

2. Soil Depletion: The amount of boron in the soil where plants are cultivated determines how readily available boron is in foods. Produce in areas with boron-deficient soils may have reduced quantities of boron, which could lead to insufficient intake.

3. Food Processing and Cooking Techniques:
Using food processing methods like refining and milling, the amount of boron in food products can be eliminated or reduced. In addition, some cooking techniques, such as boiling and using a lot of water, may cause foods to lose some of their boron content, lowering dietary intake.

4. Increased Losses: A shortage in boron may emerge from certain conditions or circumstances that cause the body to lose more boron than usual. They include disorders that impair boron absorption or usage, as well as increased perspiration, gastrointestinal distress, and vomiting.

Symptoms of Boron Deficiency

Although boron insufficiency is uncommon, a prolonged period of insufficient boron intake can have negative effects on one's health. Following are some potential signs of boron deficiency:

1. Poor Bone Health: Boron is essential for maintaining bone health, and a shortage may lead to a decrease in bone mineral density and an increase in the risk of osteoporosis. Brittle bones, an increased risk of fractures, and a slower rate of fracture healing are possible symptoms.

2. Hormonal Imbalances: Since boron is involved in the regulation of hormones, hormonal imbalances may result from a boron deficit. This can show up in women as irregular menstruation, low estrogen, and a higher chance of menopausal symptoms. Boron deficiency in men may contribute to lower testosterone levels and associated symptoms, including diminished libido, exhaustion, and weak muscles.

3. Cognitive Impairment: Boron has been associated with cognitive function, and a lack of it may affect the health of the brain and cognitive function. Poor memory, difficulties concentrating, and diminished cognitive ability are examples of symptoms.

4. Joint Pain: A lack of boron has been linked to problems with the joints, including pain, stiffness, and discomfort. This may be connected to boron's involvement in supporting joint health and the metabolism of specific substances important for joint function.

5. Poor Immune Responses: Boron supports the immune system, and its shortage may be linked to poor immunological responses. Boron shortages can lead to a reduced immune system, increased susceptibility to infections, and extended healing times.

CHAPTER 4
THE ROLE OF BORON IN HEALTH AND DISEASE

Arthritis and Joint Health

For its possible involvement in controlling arthritis, a disorder marked by joint pain and inflammation, boric acid has been researched. More studies are required to validate the findings, but research suggests that boron may reduce the symptoms of arthritis.

Boron is thought to be involved in the metabolism of substances like collagen and glycosaminoglycan's, which are essential for joint health. These elements support the cartilage's flexibility and structural integrity as it cushions the joints. Boron may improve joint health and lessen the symptoms of arthritis by boosting the synthesis and preservation of these substances.

According to certain research, boron supplements help reduce the symptoms of osteoarthritis, a prevalent kind of arthritis marked by the deterioration of joint cartilage. It has been hypothesized that boron may lessen joint discomfort, stiffness, and inflammation, resulting in increased joint function and mobility.

The research on boron's impact on arthritic conditions and joint health is, however, still in its early stages, and more research is required to determine the best doses, durations of treatment, and long-term outcomes.

Osteoporosis Prevention

Low bone density and bone tissue degeneration are the hallmarks of osteoporosis, which increases fragility and increases the risk of fractures. A healthy intake of boron may contribute to the prevention of osteoporosis and the promotion of general bone health.

Numerous procedures involving the metabolism of bones involve the element boreon. It facilitates the absorption and utilization of calcium, a mineral necessary for strong bones. Additionally, estrogen and testosterone, which are important for maintaining bone density and preventing bone loss, are affected by the presence of boreon in the body.

Boron supplementation may boost bone mineral density (BMD) and lower the risk of osteoporosis, according to a number of studies. Boron supplementation has shown promise for retaining bone mass and lowering the incidence of fractures in postmenopausal women, who are particularly vulnerable to bone loss due to hormonal changes.

While boron may benefit bone health, it should not be viewed as a stand-alone treatment for osteoporosis. This is crucial to remember. A multifaceted strategy is required to prevent osteoporosis, which includes a balanced diet high in calcium and other bone-strengthening elements, regular weight-bearing activity, optimal vitamin D levels, and avoiding behaviors that accelerate bone loss, such as smoking and binge drinking.

Menopausal Symptoms Relief

Women experience menopause as a normal biological process when they reach a specific age, usually between their late 40s and early 50s. It is characterized by a decrease in hormone production, especially estrogen, which can result in a number of symptoms and physical abnormalities. Treatment for some menopausal symptoms with boron supplements has shown success.

Women who are going through menopause may encounter symptoms like vaginal dryness, vaginal hot flashes, night sweats, mood fluctuations, and disturbed sleep. The possible advantages of boron during menopause are thought to be connected to its impact on hormone balance and levels.

The body's levels of physiologically active estrogen have been discovered to rise in the presence of the element boron, which may help lessen menopausal symptoms. Boron supplementation has demonstrated potential for reducing the frequency and intensity of hot flashes and night sweats, stabilizing mood, and reducing vaginal dryness via boosting estrogen synthesis or usage.

Even though boron may help with some menopausal symptoms, reactions can differ from person to person. The best amount and time to take boron supplements for menopause-related advantages are also still being researched. In order to evaluate whether boron supplementation is suitable for treating menopausal symptoms in your particular situation, it is advised that you speak with a healthcare practitioner.

It's also critical to keep in mind that menopause is a complicated process and that treating its symptoms fully may require a variety of strategies, such as lifestyle adjustments, hormone replacement therapy (HRT), and other treatments that are suited to each patient's needs and preferences.

We will discuss dietary boron sources, boron supplementation, and the suggested daily intake of this crucial mineral in the sections that follow.

Cognitive Function Enhancement

Memory, attention, problem-solving, and decision-making are just a few of the mental operations referred to as cognitive function. For its potential to improve brain health and boost cognitive function, boron has been studied.

According to research, the element boron may improve memory and cognitive function. It is thought to affect brain synaptic activity and neurotransmitter activity, both of which are essential for optimum cognitive function. The neurotransmitters dopamine and serotonin are among those that boron may help release and use, which means that it may enhance memory, attention, and general cognitive capacities.

The antioxidant properties of boron may also contribute to its impact on cognitive function. Cognitive function can be hampered, and age-related cognitive decline might be accelerated by oxidative stress and inflammation in the brain. Boron's capacity to lessen oxidative stress and inflammation may serve as a defense against neurological disorders and cognitive decline.

Borax has the potential to act as a neuroprotective agent and cognitive enhancer, although the precise processes by which it affects cognitive function are still under investigation. However, it is significant to highlight that boron's effects on cognitive function may differ from person to person, and further research is required to establish the best dosages and long-term benefits.

In addition to boron supplements, it's essential to lead a healthy lifestyle that includes a well-balanced diet, regular exercise, mental stimulation, stress reduction, and enough sleep to enhance cognitive performance and brain health.

The dietary sources of boron, prospective applications for boron supplements, and the suggested daily intake of this crucial mineral are all covered in the sections that follow.

Antimicrobial Properties

A putative antibacterial property of boron is its capacity to prevent the development and activity of microorganisms like bacteria, fungus, and viruses.

Although there hasn't been much research done in this area, early investigations into boron's antibacterial properties have yielded encouraging results.

The antibacterial properties of boron can be related to its capacity to damage microbial cell membranes, obstruct cellular functions, and prevent some microbes from producing particular enzymes. It has shown effectiveness against a variety of diseases, including bacteria that are immune to conventional antibiotics.

In particular, boron has demonstrated potential for preventing the growth of several bacteria, including Escherichia coli and Staphylococcus aureus, which are known to cause a variety of diseases in people. Boron has been found to have antimicrobial effects against a variety of fungi, including Candida albicans, a common source of fungal infections.

Although boron's antibacterial characteristics are intriguing, it's vital to remember that further study is required to completely comprehend their mechanisms of action, establish the best dosages, and evaluate their effectiveness in various clinical scenarios. Boron should not be used in place of recognized antimicrobial therapies or preventive measures, such as good hygiene habits and taking medication as directed.

CHAPTER 5
FOOD SOURCES OF BORON

Many meals made from plants contain naturally occurring boric acid. Following are a few typical dietary sources of boron:

1. Fruits: Many fruits contain boron, but raisins, prunes, dried apricots, peaches, and oranges have some of the highest concentrations.

2. Vegetables are yet another excellent source of boron. Vegetables with high boron content include Brussels sprouts, broccoli, spinach, kale, asparagus, and green beans.

3. Legumes: A considerable amount of boron is present in legumes such as lentils, chickpeas, soybeans, and kidney beans.

4. Nuts and Seeds: Nuts and seeds such as flaxseeds, almonds, walnuts, peanuts, and sunflower seeds are all high in boron.

5. Whole Grains: Different types of whole grains,

such as brown rice, quinoa, oats, and barley, contain boron in varied amounts.

6. Avocado: The fruit of the avocado is reputed to contain a fair quantity of boron.

7. Honey: Although the amounts may differ depending on the source, honey has been proven to contain boron

8. Grapes: Both red and green grapes have a moderate level of boron in them.

9. Apples: Apples, especially when eaten with the peel, are a good source of boron.

10. Pears: Pears are a good source of boron as well.

11. Plums: Boron is known to be present in plums, notably dried prunes.

12. Cranberries: A tart berry with some boron in it, cranberries

13. Cabbage: Green and red cabbage are both types of vegetables that contain boron.

14. Carrots: Another vegetable that contains a minor quantity of boron is the carrot.

15. Onions: Raw and cooked onions both have traces of boron in them.

16. Garlic offers a small quantity of boron and is a delicious food.

17. Celery: Boron is present in the crisp vegetable celery.

18. Sun-dried tomatoes in particular contain a tiny quantity of boron.

19. Prickly pears: Also known as cactus fruit, prickly pears have boron in them.

20. Various kinds of mushrooms, such as white button mushrooms and shiitake mushrooms, are good sources of boron.

21. Beets are a type of root vegetable that has a modest amount of boron in them.

22. Turnips: Turnips are a good source of boron, both in the root and the greens.

23. Legume sprouts: Compared to their unsprouted counterparts, sprouted legumes like lentils or mung beans may contain higher quantities of boron.

24. Raspberries are a fruit that has a minor amount of boron in them.

25. Blackberries are another fruit with a small quantity of boron, at number

26. Kiwi fruit, which contains a minor quantity of boron, is number

27. Pineapple is a tropical fruit that has a negligible amount of boron in it.

28. Watermelon is a delicious fruit that contains a negligible quantity of boron.

29. Seaweed: Kelp and wakame are two varieties of seaweed that are known to contain boron.

30. Prunes are a good source of boron and are made from dried plums.

31. Dates are tasty fruits with a moderate quantity

of boron.

32. Figs: Both fresh and dried figs have boron in them.

33. Brazil nuts are a type of nut that contains a negligible amount of boron.

34. Pistachio nuts provide a small quantity of boron, according to number

35. Sesame seeds are a seed alternative that contains boron.

CHAPTER 6
BORON SUPPLEMENTS

Creating a Brain-Healthy Environment

Depending on your age, sex, and stage of life, a different amount of boron per day may be advised. It is crucial to remember that various nations and medical organizations may have different recommendations for boron intake. Here are some suggestions for everyone:

1. The United States does not have a precise recommended dietary allowance (RDA) for boron, according to the U.S. Food and Nutrition Board of the National Academies of Sciences, Engineering, and Medicine. The following is their recommended acceptable intake (AI) level for boron, though:

Adults (including those who are pregnant or nursing): 1-3 mg daily

2. According to the European Food Safety Authority (EFSA), boron does not have a defined reference intake set forth by the agency. They have, however,

recommended a daily appropriate intake (AI) for adults of 1 mg.

Types of Boron Supplements

On the market, there are numerous varieties of boron supplements. These are the typical boron supplement forms:

1. Boron Citrate: A well-liked boron supplement is boron citrate. Boron and citric acid are combined to increase boron's bioavailability and rate of absorption in the body.

2. Boron Glycinate: Another type of boron supplement, boron glycinate mixes the mineral with the amino acid glycine. Additionally well-known for its high bioavailability is this version.

3. Boron Complexes: Complexes, including boron chelates or boron amino acid complexes, can also be found in boron supplements. Boron is bound to other substances to form these complexes, which can increase boron's stability and absorption.

4. Boron Tablets or Capsules: Boron supplements

are frequently sold as tablets or capsules. These are simple to swallow and offer a practical way to take boron supplements.

5. Boron Supplements in Liquid Form: Some boron supplements are available in liquid form, which can be consumed on its own or mixed with liquids. When comparing liquid supplements to pills or capsules, quicker absorption may be possible.

Safety Considerations

Several safety concerns should be kept in mind when supplementing with boron:

1. Recommended Dosage: It's critical to adhere to the dosage recommendations for boron supplements. Boron toxicity can develop if you consume too much of it. Respect the suggested daily consumption or the dosage that has been approved by a doctor.

2. Potential Adverse Effects: Although boron is generally regarded as safe when taken at the right levels, some people may experience adverse effects like nausea, diarrhea, or skin rashes. Stop using the boron supplement immediately and seek medical advice if you notice any negative side effects.

3. Boron supplements may interfere with some drugs, including hormone replacement therapy (HRT) and osteoporosis medications. Before beginning a boron supplement regimen, it is vital to check with your healthcare professional to be sure there are no potential drug interactions.

4. Boron supplementation has not been well researched with regard to safety during pregnancy and nursing. Avoiding high-dose boron supplements is advised during these times, and it is always preferable to speak with a healthcare provider for more specific guidance.

5. Medical disorders: Boron supplementation should be used with caution by people who have certain medical disorders, such as renal or liver disease. If you have any pre-existing medical conditions, it is crucial that you speak with a medical expert.

6. Quality and Purity: To make sure supplements are of the highest quality and purity, choose recognized brands and look for supplements that go through independent testing. This could make sure you're getting dependable and safe goods.

CHAPTER 7
POTENTIAL RISKS AND SIDE EFFECTS OF BORON

While boron is generally regarded as safe when taken in moderation, taking too much of it might have dangers and adverse effects. Here are some things to think about:

1. Boron Toxicity: Boron toxicity can result from high boron intake, particularly from supplements. Borax poisoning can cause fatigue, headaches, nausea, vomiting, diarrhea, abdominal pain, and skin rashes. Neurological problems and kidney damage are possible in severe situations. It is essential to adhere to suggested dosage recommendations and prevent overconsumption.

2. Hormonal Effects: Boron can alter the body's hormone levels. While this may help with some issues, such as menopausal symptoms, excessive consumption of boron may throw off the body's hormonal balance. Exercise caution and seek medical advice before taking boron supplements if you have a disease that makes you sensitive to hormones or if you take hormone-related medications.

3. Drug Interactions: Boron supplements may interact with some drugs, such as hormone replacement therapy (HRT) and osteoporosis treatments. The effects of boron on hormone levels and bone metabolism may affect the efficiency or security of these drugs. If you are on any drugs, it is essential to speak with a healthcare provider to find out if boron supplementation is right for you.

4. Allergic Reactions: Some people may be allergic to the element boron or some of its derivatives. After taking a boron supplement, if you develop allergic symptoms like itchiness, swelling, or trouble breathing, stop using it right away and get medical help right away.

5. Pregnancy and breastfeeding: It is not widely known whether boron supplementation is safe during pregnancy and breastfeeding. It is typically advised to steer clear of high-dose boron supplements during these times, and it is always preferable to speak with a healthcare provider for more specific guidance.

6. Pre-existing disorders: Those who already have renal, liver, or other pre-existing disorders should use caution when using boron supplements. In these circumstances, boron metabolism and removal may be impacted, which could have negative consequences. For people with underlying medical issues, consultation with a healthcare expert is crucial.

7. Digestive Problems: Some people may have gastrointestinal discomfort, such as stomach upset, indigestion, and diarrhea, as a result of excessive dosages of boron or sensitive stomachs. Starting with a lower dose and gradually increasing it if acceptable is advised.

8. Effects on Fertility: The effects of boron on male fertility have been researched. Although very high dosages of boron may have negative effects on sperm quality and fertility, low to moderate boron intake is thought to be safe. Men who are trying to get pregnant should use caution and talk to a doctor before using boron supplements.

9. Blood Clotting: Boron can interfere with the body's natural blood clotting processes. When using boron supplements, people who are taking blood-thinning medications like warfarin or who have bleeding disorders should exercise caution because it may increase the risk of bleeding. To examine potential interactions, it is crucial to speak with a healthcare expert.

10. Effect on Thyroid Function: According to some research, consuming too much boron may impair thyroid function by preventing thyroid hormones from working properly. Boron supplements should only be taken under the supervision of a healthcare provider and with caution by people with thyroid conditions or those using thyroid drugs.

11. Electrolyte Imbalance: High amounts of boron can throw off the equilibrium of several electrolytes, like calcium, magnesium, and potassium, in the body. People who suffer from particular medical ailments, such as kidney illness or cardiac issues, may be affected by this. For people with underlying illnesses, expert medical advice is crucial.

12. Reduced Nutrient Absorption: Too much boron can prevent the body from absorbing and using other important minerals like calcium and magnesium. This might have an effect on nutrition and total mineral balance. A balanced diet and avoiding consuming too much boron can help reduce this risk.

CONCLUSION

In conclusion, the trace mineral boron has a number of significant functions in the human body. Boron has been discovered to have a number of positive impacts on health and wellbeing, despite the fact that it is only needed in modest amounts. By improving calcium metabolism and encouraging the development of robust bones, it enhances bone health. By taking part in the metabolism of estrogen, testosterone, and vitamin D, boron also helps regulate hormones.

Additionally, boron has been linked to enhanced memory and cognitive function in the brain. Additionally, it might provide immune system support, bolstering the body's defenses against illnesses and infections. Because of its anti-inflammatory effects, boron is advantageous for treating diseases like arthritis and maintaining joint health.

Additionally, boron has been linked to the prevention of osteoporosis, especially in postmenopausal women, as it helps to preserve bone density and lowers the incidence of fractures. By adjusting hormone levels, it can ease menopausal symptoms, including hot flashes and mood swings.

It has been found that boron has a beneficial effect on cognitive function, suggesting that it may improve learning, memory, and attention. Additionally, boron demonstrates antibacterial qualities that may help in the battle against specific bacteria and fungi.

Although boron is naturally found in a variety of foods, such as fruits, vegetables, nuts, and legumes, supplementation may be warranted in some circumstances. Toxicology, hormone imbalance, digestive problems, worries about fertility, and drug interactions are just a few of the potential hazards and side effects of consuming too much boron.

Following the suggested daily consumption recommendations and speaking with a medical professional or qualified dietician are crucial for ensuring the safe and efficient use of boron. Based on your medical history, current medications, and unique circumstances, they can evaluate your particular needs, identify any risks, and offer you individualized guidance.

When thinking about boron supplements, it's crucial to pick reliable companies that go through independent testing to guarantee quality and purity. You can reduce the chance of consuming contaminated or subpar products by doing this.